THE

SLEEP SOLUTION

How to Correct Your Sleep With Head-To-Toe Healing

Dr. Kevin Reese

www.DRKEVINREESE.com

The Sleep Solution

Seven Thirty Enterprises LLC

ISBN: 979-8-9860807-7-2

Copyright © 2025

No information in this book is intended as a substitute for the medical advice of a licensed physician. Kevin Reese, PhD, PAS, INHC, DS is NOT a licensed physician. Kevin Reese is a doctor of philosophy (phd) and is known as a head to toe healer who educates others on the topic of health and wellness.

Dr. Reese does not diagnose, treat or cure diseases, instead he gives assessments, provides education and gives recommendations based on the belief that the human body is divinely designed to heal itself.

You should check with your licensed primary care physician anytime you change diet or exercise. You should also seek medical care if you have an infection, a new injury or are in urgent need of attention.

Although the author and publisher have made every effort to ensure that the information in this book was correct at press time, the author and publisher do not assume and hereby disclaim any liability to any party for any loss, damage, or disruptions caused by errors or omissions, whether such errors or omissions result from negligence or any other cause.

The writings in this book are meant for educational purposes. If you take any advice from this book, you do so at your own discretion.

Table of Contents

THE RECHARGING

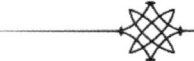

So you're not sleeping well, huh?

How long has this been happening?

I've been there. I know what it's like. It sucks!

You're a part of the "walking dead."

You already know what I'm about to tell you; this "walking dead" zone will create major fear and frustration in your life.

There's so many nerdy influencers out there on youtube teaching the science of sleep. They'll tell you that sleep is typically divided into two main stages, rapid eye movement (REM) sleep and non-REM (NREM) sleep. NREM sleep consists of four progressively deeper stages, while REM sleep is characterized by rapid eye movements, increased brain activity, and vivid dreaming.

The nerds will also tell you to get some fancy watch that will keep track of your deep sleep (SWS). SWS is a deep sleep stage characterized by slow brain waves, reduced muscle activity, and minimal dreaming. It's also known as the "orthodox phase" of sleep. According to scientists, adults need around 1.5 - 2 hours of deep sleep per night. Many of them say that deep sleep is the key to good rest.

My approach is to not measure anything.

Don't listen to the nerds. Knowledge is best on a macro level, not a micro level.

From my viewpoint, measuring will only create paranoia and phobias. I don't want you to worry about science. I don't even want you to worry about sleep. I want you to accept the sleepless night without frustration.

Truly I tell you, the less you worry, the better you will sleep.

Do you understand what I have just told you?

It's deep.

It's spiritual.

I would also like to encourage you to stay away from the term "Insomnia." This is just another dis-ease label the Medical Monopoly uses to create cash flow. You don't have a dis-ease, you have trouble sleeping. Take "insomnia" out of your language for good.

All you need to know is that sleep is a process of recharging your batteries so you can operate in the world the next day. We need sleep because being a part of the "walking dead" will alter your day. Life is ridiculously harder with a lack of sleep.

You're not the only one by any means as the sleep economy is a big business. Think about how many mattress commercials you've seen in your lifetime. How about pillow infomercials? Now add in the legal drugs, medical devices, sleep clinics and even natural sleep aids. The sleep economy was reported to bring in $64 Billion in the year 2023. Of course, it's going to keep growing due to the increasing prevalence of sleep deprivation.

We have an epidemic. The World Health Organization (WHO) says that two-thirds of adults sleep less than eight hours per night. In the United States, the CDC estimates that 50 to 70 million adults have chronic sleep disorders.

In this book, I'm going to tell you the solution to your sleeping issue.

Like anything I teach, it takes work.

Are you OK with putting in some work?

If you don't, you will stay in the "walking dead" zone.

It's your choice.

THE SUBCONSCIOUS MIND

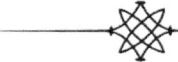

Inside your skull is a brain. That brain is essentially an on-board computer. It controls the rest of your body because it's attached to your spine. The spine is like a circuit breaker that sends signals to the rest of the body. This is called your nervous system.

Your brain has an executive part that is very conscious. This executive makes decisions and solves problems. The executive is like the adult in the room and tells you when to brush your teeth, take a left turn at the stop sign, evaluate a business deal, etcetera.

Underneath the adult (executive) there is a powerful database system that stores your programming which is your beliefs, your values, your deeper memories, your traumas, your habits, your patterns and your personality. Because this processing system happens unconsciously it is typically referred to as the subconscious mind.

For example, the habit of biting your nails comes from the subconscious mind. The way you laugh comes from the subconscious mind. The angry reaction you have when your mother says "that thing" comes from the subconscious mind. Your fear of certain animals comes from the subconscious mind. Your belief that you're not good enough comes from the subconscious mind. Your PTSD comes from the subconscious mind. And most certainly, your sleeping patterns come from the subconscious mind.

Guess what? Your healing also comes from the subconscious mind. It essentially governs over your 11 bodily systems. When you're sleeping the subconscious mind repairs your cells, cleans out toxins, fights inflammation and so much more.

The good news is that you can reprogram the subconscious mind. The bad news is that it takes a lot of time and it's very tedious. This is what I've referred to in my books, videos and seminars as mindfulness training. Mindfulness training is ⅓ of the practice of HEAD TO TOE HEALING.

In order to reprogram the subconscious mind we have to understand the innocence of this part of your computer. The subconscious mind is almost like a camera. It just records and picks things up around it without an opinion. Whatever it records goes into the database (like a digital cloud) and gets stored. That data can be rerun at any time which means your thoughts could go to that recording while you're driving or while you're sleeping.

Because the subconscious mind is so innocent, the best way to work with it is to use the analogy of a child, specifically, a 2 year old child who likes to get into a little trouble. Now that you know that you have an inner child, your job, as an adult, is to nurture and console it as much as possible. That's really all you can do because you can not control what data it spits out.

After you watch your inner child for a few weeks you will notice that it becomes scared, angry, guilty, obsessed, etcetera. Your "little you" goes through an array of thoughts and feelings and it's your job, as the adult, to talk very kindly and warmly to it.

As you talk kindly and warmly to your inner child, remember that your subconscious mind can have a great impact on your entire body. Therefore, you can ask for help. You can ask to relieve the pain in your left knee, you can ask to stop obsessing over your ex boyfriend. You can ask to sleep better. The list goes on.

Will the inner child help right away? No! It takes time. You have neglected your inner child for so long that it's going to be a little hesitant at first. You've been a "deadbeat" parent and your inner child needs to warm up to you. It needs to trust you. Prove yourself to your "little you." Be patient. Talk to your inner child one hundred times per day if you have to.

You can give your inner child a pet name so that your talking is more warm. You simply put your left hand on your heart and then your right hand over your left hand. Now you can caress your hand with warmth and love and close your eyes. Rubbing your hand for about ten seconds with your eyes closed will put you into the vibration of compassion. Then you talk to your inner child. It doesn't have to be long.

The framework is…

1-   Acknowledge the issue

2-   Take responsibility

3-   Ask for help

4-   Show appreciation for helping

5-   Give the assurance of love and safety

Example...

1-   Baby, I'm sorry that your not sleeping well tonight

2-   Please forgive me for whatever I've done to cause this situation

3-   I ask you to shut this body down so we can get good rest

4-   Thank you so much for helping with this sleep

5-   I love you so much and I'm here for you

You can play around with your sentences but you want to keep the general framework which is taking responsibility and showing love.

You must keep petitioning your inner child as much as possible. The more you talk, the more you will create a connection with your subconscious mind which inturn will start working in your favor. Your inner child is there to help you.

It's also significant to note that this does not replace prayer to God. If you're a Godly person, please continue to pray. It's important to understand that God created you and the computer in your skull. So by talking to your subconscious mind God will be proud of you because you're using the gifts and tools that he has given you. You see, praying to God is outward, whereas talking to your inner child is inward. One is apples and one is oranges, but both fruits are in the same orchard.

Now, get to work. Don't hesitate, you must start building this connection ASAP.

CIRCADIAN RHYTHM

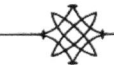

If you eat lunch everyday at 1pm your body is going to expect food everyday at 1pm. If you have a bowel movement every morning at 6am your body will expect to have a bowel movement everyday at 6am. If you go to bed every night at 9pm your body will expect to go to bed every night at 9pm. This is the circadian rhythm. It's a biological schedule that your body adapts to and follows.

Have you ever known someone who has weird sleeping habits? Perhaps they go to sleep at 2am every night and sleep half the day away. Now they can't have a normal lifestyle. Some people even sleep in shifts. That's right, they sleep for 3 or 4 hours and then wake up, do stuff, and go back to sleep for 3 or 4 hours. Some people sleep very little and then make it up with a long nap during the day. No matter how weird the sleeping pattern is, it's running off a subconscious program that has been installed.

Now, If you break the circadian rhythm once or twice, the body will be like "what the heck are you doing?" But it won't be that big of a deal. If you start to constantly change your schedule, the inner child will react in a big way. You may experience some fear because your "little you" is going to say, "Why are you changing!? I thought we were all set."

Your circadian rhythm will change for one of two reasons. (1) Your situation and or environment is changing so you're going with the flow. (2) You're voluntarily changing your schedule because you want to improve your life.

Sometimes you can't control your situation or environment so you do have to go with the flow, however, hopefully you change your circadian rhythm because you wish to improve your life. Perhaps you've discovered that you're not living correctly and now is the time for change.

In order to reprogram the schedule you must reprogram your subconscious mind for the subconscious mind connects to your spine and your spine controls the rest of your body. In order to wrap your hands around the subconscious mind, we must use the metaphor of a child. To make this easier, visualize your 2 year old self. It just so happens that your "little you" has tremendous power over your body. Your 2 year old self can be your ally or your enemy. It's your choice.

Your first step is to write down the schedule that you want to have. Eating times, sleeping times, bowel movement times, exercise times, etcetera. Then you have to follow the schedule so that you can begin to retrain the body. While you go through this retraining, you must constantly talk to your inner child and nurture it so that the backlash isn't harsh.

Simply place your left hand on your heart and then put your right hand on top of your left hand. Now caress the hand as if you were hugging your 2 year old self and close your eyes. You can say something like, "Baby, don't worry about the change in schedule. I'm going to make our lives better. Don't be scared, I'll take care of everything. I love you."

It's very key that you always end your statements with "I love you."

You can also be very specific when you talk to your inner child. You can say, "Darling, we are going to go to bed at 9pm tonight and we are going to sleep until 5am. We are going to wake up feeling fresh and rested. It's going to be very satisfying. Then we will drink some water, do some exercises and have our morning bowel elimination. Please help me do this. Thank you and I love you."

Now you have to give your subconscious mind some help to perform the reprograming. This will be done through light exposure. It's important to understand that when light enters the eye, the brain stops producing melatonin, a hormone that helps with sleep. That said, an hour before bed you should turn off as many lights as possible and most certainly not look at your smartphone or tablet. Your bedroom, of course, should be pitch black. You may even wish to consider a sleep mask.

Now, when you wake up you do the opposite. You need to get into as much light as possible. That's going to be your phone, your tablet, your computer, all the lights in the house, etcetera. The best light of course is the sun, so open the curtains and or go outside if the sun is up and it's not cold. Get as much light as you can.

Another cheat code on resetting your circadian rhythm is the water chug. I've been having clients do this for 15 years and it works. Prepare a glass of water (at least 8 oz) with a pinch of celtic sea salt and have it nearby. I personally keep mine in my office which is next to my bedroom. Somewhere inside the first 10 minutes of waking up, chug that water. When I say chug, I mean it literally, don't sip. Pretend you're a freshman in college and you're at a beer party. Chug, chug, chug! Not only will the salt water chug help reprogram your circadian rhythm but it will hydrate you, wake up your digestive system and promote a run to the toilet.

If you want to reprogram your circadian rhythm it's going to take discipline and courage. It can be a little tedious, but it will be completed for those that are serious about my teachings.

BLUE BOOK BONUS

I recorded a whole album of bedtime stories for you. Try them as you're going to sleep.

They're available on all streaming platforms such as spotify, apple music or youtube music.

Access yours: https://www.drkevinreese.com/voice

NUTRITION

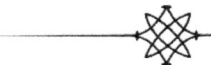

Your sleep is affected by your biochemistry. The raw material that makes up your biochemistry is called nutrition. You see, there's 90 essential nutrients that the body needs daily. Essential means that the nutrients are not made by the body, so they need to be imported.

Unfortunately, it's not possible to import these nutrients through food due to soil depletion. That's right, our soil is not what it used to be because of corporate farming and the damming of rivers. So something as simple as an apple was healthier 200 years ago than it is now.

The best way to get around this soil issue is to supplement. In recent years supplements such as sea moss and moringa have become popular. While they both can help you, they are not lab tested which means you don't know how much nutrition is actually in it. That's why I teach my people to buy certain lab tested supplements in my virtual learning membership.

However, even the best supplements still need to be absorbed into your bloodstream. This is why I teach my people to get off of the poor four foods (gluten, oils, fried and fake) as soon as possible. These foods not only block absorption, but they also create inflammation. This means the body will have to do more repair work and overcompensate, hence hurting your sleep.

The other factor in your diet is sugar. Although sugar is not part of the poor four foods it can still be one of the causes of sleep issues. Sugar can keep you up at night because consuming it causes a rapid spike in blood sugar levels, which then triggers the release of insulin, leading to a subsequent drop in blood sugar that can leave you feeling alert and energized. Lowering your carbohydrates (sugar) to around 200 MG per day could be a game changer to your sleep quality.

Caffeine is also not part of the poor four foods but can affect your sleeping greatly. It's probably the number one stimulant on earth and certainly the biggest addiction. It's found in colored tea, coffee, and cacao plants. Yes, it's known to improve alertness and response time but it's also known to wreak havoc on your nervous system. Getting off of caffeine would be a wise move for anyone that has sleeping issues. It's common sense.

It's important to note that the human body only has two macronutrient fuel sources. It's carbohydrates and fat. So whichever one is lower the other must come up higher. If you bring your carbs lower, then fats like eggs, avocado, beef and butter must come up higher. Protein is not a fuel source, so lean meats won't help if you lower your carbs.

Don't underestimate nutrition on the micro level. It's very possible that someone is not sleeping because of a simple nutritional deficiency of the 90 essential nutrients. You might be surprised to know that each nutritional deficiency can cause up to 10 symptoms. That means you can have up to 900 symptoms from a lack of nutrition.

When it comes to sleep, the most needed nutrient in the human body is calcium. Calcium helps regulate the sleep-wake cycle by influencing the activity of neurons involved in sleep. This doesn't mean go to the store and buy up calcium. Nutrition is more complicated than that as ratios are involved. Calcium needs to be in alignment with zinc, magnesium, phosphorus, copper, etcetera to work properly. Again, this is why buying the right supplements that are formulated well is important.

Many people are on the magnesium wave now and take doses of magnesium glycinate to help their sleep. This can help at first, but the body will still be looking for 89 other nutrients.

When it comes to your biochemistry you have a hormone that is secreted from your adrenal glands called cortisol. It's known as the stress hormone which creates the infamous "fight or flight" response in the body. Needless to say, stressed out people have higher levels of cortisol in their body which most certainly would disrupt sleep patterns.

A lower carb and higher fat diet that is free of the poor four foods should help cortisol levels. However, sometimes that's not enough. In my virtual learning membership, I teach my people to take an amino acid called L-theanine which relaxes your nervous system and balances cortisol levels. There's also herbal formulas I teach that act as cortisol managers right before bedtime.

I like to have my students take these cortisol managers for only a few months to balance their hormones and then drop formulas for good. I don't feel that there is a need to "take something" nightly before bed. I don't want you to be reliant on anything because in the long run, it will cause superstition, phobias and paranoia.

POSTURE

(MUSCULOSKELETAL ALIGNMENT)

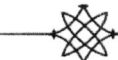

Could you not be sleeping because of a compressed nerve? Yes!

There are 7 trillion nerves in the human body. It's a divinely designed electrical system that delivers signals to your organs, glands and tissues to create bodily functions. One of those functions is obviously sleep.

In my book, REVERSE THE CAUSE, I lay out the 7 root causes to dis-ease. One of those causes is muscle dysfunction. You see, when your muscles are out of alignment, they pull your bones into odd positions. In doing so, they can compress the nerves which in turn will either alter bodily function and or create pain.

A pinched nerve in the neck (cervical spine) is the most common area that can significantly affect sleep, as it can cause pain and discomfort that worsens when lying down. The vagus nerve which runs from the brain to the large intestine is a part of your autonomic nervous system and helps reduce stress and promotes relaxation. When this nerve is compressed, your sleep can be disrupted in a major way.

So while most people will run to the chiropractor or osteopath to release a nerve for short-term relief we use the practice of HEAD TO TOE HEALING to achieve long lasting reversals of causes. That said, ⅓ of HEAD TO TOE HEALING is postural alignment therapy (PAT) to get the muscles back into alignment. PAT needs to be performed daily and is to your muscles what brushing and flossing is to your mouth.

Some of my students receive relief from their compressed nerves in just a day and some in a full year, it just depends on how wound up your muscles are.

I have put together a PAT sleep routine for you. I urge you to take this seriously and commit to the following plan:

1. Perform the routine twice daily — once in the morning and once in the evening — for two weeks straight. Then stop. This routine is NOT designed to be all the time, just for 2 weeks.

2. If you're interested in more PAT (postural alignment therapy), you can join my virtual learning membership and come to our live classes.

After completing your PAT session, it's essential to follow up with two activities:

- Drink water: Hydration is crucial for supporting your body's healing process.

- Go for a walk: Walking helps "activate" the muscles you've just worked on during therapy.

If you don't have time for a full walk, simply move around the room where you performed the therapy. Think of this as "walking it off." PAT enhances muscle functionality, and walking integrates these changes into your daily movement patterns.

BLUE BOOK BONUS

I made a sleep rescue program for you. It contains supplement recommendations, a postural alignment therapy routine and inner child work.

It's available inside the Blue Book Bonus Trainings.

Access yours for FREE: www.drkevinreese.com/bluebonus

CLIMATE CONTROL

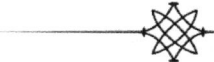

You have to control your climate if you want to sleep well. You see, your subconscious mind (inner child) lowers your internal temperature and releases sleep hormones as it prepares your body for sleep. Therefore, if you make your room cold it's a "cheat-code" to reach this state of sleep. It also programs your circadian rhythm and lets your inner child know that it's sleep time.

You need your room between 60 and 65 degrees fahrenheit. Therefore, an hour or two before bedtime, you should make sure your room is getting colder. Many people don't like the cold. My response to them is, "Do you want to sleep well?" It doesn't have to be so cold that you're shaking, it just needs to be cold enough to get under those covers and feel nice and toasty. You can add a microfiber blanket to put on top of what you already have. You will appreciate the sheets and covers so much more, especially if you're naked.

Using myself as an example, I always keep an air conditioner in my bedroom window. Yes, even in the New England winter. Certainly, the a/c unit breaks down faster but I simply invest in a new one every two years. I always make sure it has a regulating thermostat on it so if the temperature of the room goes above 65 degrees, it turns on. This allows me to control my climate whereas the rest of the house might have different temperatures. If you live with people there might be a tussle for the thermostat, but you can control your room.

Speaking of temperature, you want to make sure you don't eat spicy food for dinner. Spicy foods can run through your digestive system very slowly and heat you up even three hours after you eat it. This can be foods like cayenne pepper, garlic, onions, pepperoni, etcetera.

Stay cool.

CHRONIC PAIN

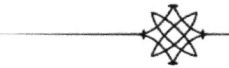

Chronic pain is a major reason why many people don't sleep well. Whether it's back pain, knee pain, neck pain, migraines or sciatica, the discomfort can lead to a real miserable state.

If you're in this much pain, you must first go to your inner child (subconscious mind) to calm it down. You must say…

"Baby, I'm sorry that this body is hurting right now. Please forgive me for whatever I've done to contribute to this pain. I'm asking you to kindly heal this body internally while I work on the external side. Thank you for doing this and I love you."

OK, so you just promised your inner child that you would take care of it externally. Now, you must live up to the promise.

Step 1: Get off the poor four foods (gluten, oils, fried and fake)

Step 2: Lay in static back for 20 minutes per day

Step 3: Read my books and or spend time in my educational library on my website

Step 4: Order your HEAD TO TOE Analysis to find the root causes to your symptoms

Step 5: Join my virtual learning membership and start practicing, HEAD TO TOE HEALING

It's no accident that we have the most healing results ever recorded on video. It would take you six hours or more to watch every person testifying to their pain disappearing.

If you read my book, MEDICAL MONOPOLY then you know that if you go to the white coats, they will lead you down a very dark path that can lead to despair and hopelessness.

Their only solution is drugs, injections and surgeries. This $1.6 trillion dollar empire is not trained to heal you, they are trained to treat symptoms, stabilize you and manage your pain. This elaborate strategy keeps you in a vicious cycle that creates cash flow.

You don't have to live in this misery.

The practice of HEAD TO TOE HEALING is the answer.

THE POOR FOUR FEARS

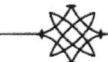

In my book, THE ANXIETY ANSWER, I talk about the poor four fears.

1-   Embarrassment

2-   Drastic Change

3-   Insanity

4-   Death

When it comes to sleep, embarrassment can show up in your dreams. The inner child hates being embarrassed. This could be a dream of you showing up to school naked or being on stage while people laugh at you. However, the real embarrassment is going to work the next day in the "walking dead" zone from sleep deprivation. The fear of embarrassment from not sleeping could snowball and create paranoia.

Drastic change could play a factor in sleep deprivation because you're worried about this big change that's happening in your life. Perhaps you're getting divorced, or you're having a baby or you're moving.

I'm a good sleeper, but when I moved a few years back, I started having trouble sleeping again. Thank God I knew the knowledge I'm sharing with you in this book because I was able to handle it. I knew that my inner child was scared and overwhelmed. I took care of little Kevin and was sleeping well again in a few days.

The third fear is insanity. This is a big factor because when you don't sleep, you start to feel insane. You start to feel like you're going crazy. You're not cognitively all there and you feel off. In fact, someone that doesn't sleep well on a normal basis almost mirrors the symptoms of an alcoholic. They can slur their words, they can make a lot of errors, they can be clumsy and they certainly lack short term memory. This can make you ponder, "Am I going insane?"

And the last fear is huge when it comes to not sleeping, and that's death. Losing consciousness is not something most people like. It's a loss of control. Passing out and losing consciousness is as close to death as you can get.

Do you remember the fear on Wendy Williams' face when she passed out on national TV? How about when you go under for a surgery? The truth is, every night we pass out, we just don't have the mindset of passing out. Instead we call it a different word called, sleep. It's like we die every single night only to be reborn again in the morning.

Not only would overcoming the four fears be good for your sleep, but it would be great for your life. So what you have to do is establish that relationship with your inner child (subconscious mind) and talk through these fears constantly. Be tedious about it. If you have spare time during the day, take ten minutes to nurture and consol your inner child on all four fears.

Example...

You simply put your left hand on your heart and then your right hand over your left hand. Now you can caress your hand with warmth and love and close your eyes. Rubbing your hand for about ten seconds with your eyes closed will put you into the vibration of compassion. Then you talk to your inner child. It doesn't have to be long as 30 seconds can be enough.

1- 	 *Baby, I'm sorry that your scared of _____ (drastic change)*

2- 	 *Please forgive me for whatever I've done to cause this situation*

3- 	 *You don't have to worry about anything because I'm going to make sure that we have food, water and shelter. You're safe. I need you to let go of this fear and help me get good sleep so I can feel refreshed in the morning. We're a team. You shut this body down for sleep and I'll take care of you.*

4- 	 *Thank you so much for being here with me and doing this for me.*

5- 	 *I love you. Everything is going to be OK.*

It's important to note that if you're really scared, you can talk to your inner child for longer. You could just freestyle it and really dig deep. You could give yourself a hug with both hands and really nurture yourself. Just gauge the situation and the level that you're at. Your inner child loves to be reassured that everything is going to be OK.

BLUE BOOK BONUS

I recorded a whole album of sleep meditations for you. Try one every night.

They're available on all streaming platforms such as spotify, apple music or youtube music.

Access yours: https://www.drkevinreese.com/voice

FEAR OF DEATH

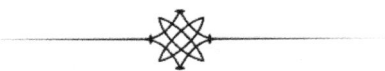

A great poet named Nasir Jones once said, "Sleep is the cousin of death."

Have you ever been around someone that's sleeping? I'm sure you have. They have no idea what's going on in the room, they're out, they're gone.

When you really ponder on the nature of sleep it's fascinating. You actually lose consciousness but the 11 systems of your body keep working. Not only are you alive and well, but your body is regenerating!

It's not talked about often, but so many people around the world have trouble sleeping because they are scared of dying. You see, sleep and death both are an act of losing consciousness. The major difference is that in sleep you have to surrender to it whereas in death you are forced into it.

Surrender is the key word here. You may view surrender as a negative word, but from a spiritual aspect it's powerful. It's letting go and letting God. It's having trust that you're going to be OK so you stop resisting.

You may not like the feeling of losing consciousness so you resist it. Your inner child (subconscious mind) does not like the feeling of being knocked out. This action is too close for comfort. It's on the edge of losing everything. Perhaps you don't want to lose your lifestyle, your children, your house, your career, your christmas parties, etcetera.

There is a deep attachment to the illusion of material life, which is coming from the computer in your skull which is pumping out an algorithm of programming.

Truly I tell you, this programing is not you. The real you is the one that is actually watching that programming. The "watcher" is an awareness which is not of this material world. Knowing this truth is powerful and can help you let go of this life.

The acceptance and appreciation of your death is a very great moment in your life's journey. Some people have to go through tough times to come to this moment. For me, I had to go through a spiritual event called, DARK NIGHT OF THE SOUL. This event lasted 7 months for me. I slept well when it was over.

Surrender.

DREAMS

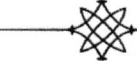

It's perfectly normal to have a vivid dream right before you wake up in the morning, however, some people dream a lot throughout the night. Perhaps you remember every detail. Truth be told, if you're dreaming that much and remembering the dream, you're obviously not getting quality sleep.

It's the same thing with daydreaming. If you're driving down the road and you're daydreaming about that thing that happened to you when you were 12 years old, you're not paying attention to the road as well as you could be.

When the inner child (subconscious mind) is babbling it's simply distracting you from whatever you're doing, sleep included. It's easy to get stuck in the movie of your mind.

It's best to continuously nurture and console your inner child when you're awake. Not only does this cleanse the data in the subconscious mind but it also helps you be aware that you are not those thoughts. You are something else that is experiencing those thoughts. It's a movie that you are watching.

When you're sleep dreaming it's a signal that your inner child needs to be nurtured and consoled more. Your "little you" is trying to tell you something. For example, if you keep dreaming about being in high school and you're 20 years removed from graduation day, perhaps your inner child is holding on to some drama that happened to you in that period of your life. Maybe it's time to clean that up.

If you're dreaming about your husband cheating on you with the hot neighbor down the street, maybe your inner child is insecure about your relationship. Perhaps it's time to clean that up.

If you keep dreaming about some mythical creature that keeps chasing you through the woods, maybe your inner child is afraid of something happening in your life right now. Let's clean that up.

If you keep dreaming about forgetting to pick your child up at school, perhaps you're feeling scared about being a competent parent. Let's cleanse.

Again, put your left hand on your heart and your right hand over the hand so you can gently rub. If you need to get in your compassionate zone, simply rub your hand with your eyes closed for about ten seconds. Then talk to your inner child lovingly…

"Baby, I'm sorry you're feeling this way (you can be descriptive here).

Please forgive me for whatever I've done to cause this.

I know that you can let go of it so it doesn't bother us anymore.

Thank you for bringing this up so we can clean it up.

I love you."

Your dreams are markers of what you need to work on. Remember, there is a two year old child in you that needs nurturing and consoling and it's on you, the adult, to handle this. If you continue to do this on a serious basis, you will start to release emotional baggage and you will reprogram your mind. The dreams will eventually fade away and you will get deeper sleep.

WAKE UP ROUTINE

Do you wake up in the middle of the night? It can be frustrating. You just want to sleep all the way through but for some reason, you're up. It happens.

The first thing you want to do is roll over into a new position and give it five minutes and see if you fall back asleep.

If you don't fall back asleep, then you need to get out of bed and go to another room of the house. This change in energy will be good for your inner child. If you have a downstairs, walking down the stairs would be ideal. Of course, keep things as dark as possible.

Once you get there you need to petition your inner child. First, ask yourself, is your inner child scared, angry, guilty, obsessed with a project? What data is pumping out? Once you identify that, you can be specific with your petition framework.

Put your left hand on your heart and then your right hand over your left hand. Now you can caress your hand with warmth and love and close your eyes. Rubbing your hand for about ten seconds with your eyes closed will put you into the vibration of compassion.

Baby, I'm sorry that you're worried about your job interview tomorrow.

Please forgive me for whatever I've done to cause you to be scared.

I ask you to shut this body down so we can get good rest.

Thank you so much for helping with this sleep.

I love you so much and I'm here for you. Everything is going to be OK.

Next, you want to perform walking meditation. You're going to simply walk from wall to wall in the room very slowly. Using the unlimited power of your mind, place your awareness into your feet and feel every step. Feel the heel of the foot and the ball of the foot hitting the floor. Walk slow. If your mind wanders in another direction, very simply bring your attention back to your feet. You can do this wall-to-wall walk about 10 times.

Then, petition your inner child again. Put your left hand on your heart and then your right hand over your left hand. Now you can caress your hand with warmth and love and close your eyes. Rubbing your hand for about ten seconds with your eyes closed will put you into the vibration of compassion.

Baby, I'm sorry that you're worried about your job interview tomorrow.

Please forgive me for whatever I've done to cause you to be scared.

I ask you to shut this body down so we can get good rest.

Thank you so much for helping with this sleep.

I love you so much and I'm here for you. Everything is going to be OK.

Now, slowly walk back to bed and get under the covers. Close your eyes, take a deep breath and see what happens. If you're still having trouble. Go back to the other room and repeat.

If you absolutely can't fall asleep, watch television and lay down. Be kind to yourself and have acceptance that this isn't your night. It's OK.

Just let go.

VISUALIZE YOUR SLEEP

You can get the result that you want by using the unlimited power of your mind to visualize what you want. So in this case, you want to visualize yourself sleeping real comfortably and soundly.

During the day, visualize yourself looking down at yourself while you're sleeping in your bed. Think of it like a scene in a movie. You're at such peace. Make this scene last a good 15 seconds in your mind.

Now I want you to visualize yourself being congratulated the next day by someone else who is genuinely happy that you told them you got great sleep last night. You can visualize me if you'd like, I'm sure you've seen plenty of my videos. Again, make this scene a good 15 seconds in your mind.

Do your best to feel an emotion while you visualize both scenes. How do you feel? Are you happy? Are you proud of yourself? Smile.

You can take the scene even further. Imagine that we are at my annual seminar and you say, "Hey Dr. Reese, I need to tell you that I'm finally sleeping well." I smile and reply, "That's amazing ____(your name), I'm so happy for you. How has your life improved from this sleep change?" You reply, "I am _____(fill in the perks). I'm smiling from ear to ear and I'm like, "That's amazing. You look great and your energy is great. I'm proud of you. Keep up the good work."

You don't have to use me in your visualization, you can use your mom, dad, son, daughter, best friend, etcetera. Who would be very happy for you?

Now run this visualization two times every day for 6 weeks straight. The most powerful time to do it is as you're dozing off to sleep. That's when you can super download to the subconscious mind (inner child).

Remember, your inner child (subconscious mind) is awake while you're sleeping. It's the executive part (the adult) of the mind that goes to sleep and becomes silent. Your inner child is still up and working on your body.

BLUE BOOK BONUS

I invite you to read or listen to my entire book collection.

The red book, *Medical Monopoly*, and the green book, *Head-To-Toe Healing*, are the most essential. Together, they complement each other and form the foundation of a new healthcare system designed for your overall wellbeing.

Check it out: https://www.drkevinreese.com/books

SLEEP SUPERSTITIONS

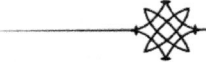

Sleep Position

Laying on your back with your head not propped up too much is the best way to sleep. This is because your spine is flatted out and your body has a chance to be in alignment while sleeping. However, it is not necessary.

Sleep is so important that you should sleep however you can. I would rather you get 8 hours in the fetal position than 2 hours on your back. Sleep in whatever position that makes you comfortable. This is why we do PAT (postural alignment therapy) in my virtual learning membership. PAT is to your muscles what brushing and flossing is to your teeth. Your muscles need to be maintained daily. I teach my people to perform cats & dogs to realign the spine first thing after getting out of bed.

Exercise Helps

I once heard a wise man say that if you've having trouble sleeping, just go for a run until you're exhausted. I believe this to be true. The more you exert yourself, the more tired you will be at day's end. However, a run isn't necessary. Getting 15,000 steps per day should do it. These days, your phone keeps track. I suggest making this a new habit. Getting your steps is healthy on an overall level anyway.

Getting 8 Hours of Sleep

Science says that adults need 8 hours of sleep. It's not true. It really depends on the person and their personality type. I know of some high level executives and entrepreneurs that sleep 4 or 5 hours a night and they operate really well in the world. Personally, I thrive off 8 or 9 hours. If I were to get 4 or 5 hours, I would feel it. It's interesting to note that historical geniuses like Nicola Tesla, Thomas Edison and Leonardo Da Vinci were known to not sleep through the night. Instead they took 20 minute naps every two hours. I don't recommend this, but it just shows you what's possible. Tesla lived until 86, Edison until 84 and Da Vinci until 67.

Fear of No Sleep

Pulling an involuntary all-nighter can be terrifying and frustrating but please understand that the body will shut down and sleep. The body doesn't stay up that long. Two straight days is usually about where it will conk out. Some people have gone for 3 or 4 days and experienced hallucinations but typically, it will rest. There's no way around it, the body will sleep. So you should always trust that it will shut down and force you into sleep. This is where petitioning the inner child is key. Talk to it and settle down the fear. You're going to be OK.

The Inner Child Remembers

It does. If you have a sleepless night on a Monday but sleep great for the rest of the week, you could have another sleepless night the following Monday. The inner child likes to play games with patterns. It's on you, the adult, to recognize this and petition your "little you."

EMF

In recent years, it's been reported that EMF (electromagnetic fields) is greatly affecting us. I don't disagree. There's so many devices and WiFi that it's got to be a factor in our overall health. It's been said that EMF can affect sleep quality. Some people suggest turning off WiFi at night before bed. It can't hurt. However, you either have to live alone or have an entire family on board with the understanding. I personally do not turn my WiFi off. However, I never sleep with my phone in the room. I always have it in the next room. I also go to sleep with the TV on, but I put an hour timer on it. So yes, I'm getting some EMF, but I sleep great 90% of the time.

Television

Many people tell you to not have a TV in your room. I say, get it how you can. Sometimes the inner child is calmed down by watching some useless TV right before bed. This can help you doze off. I would just suggest putting a timer on the TV so it's not on all night.

Background Noise

Some say that you need silence to sleep. Hogwash. Background noise can certainly help. It could be the natural sounds of a waterfall or a forest or it could be specifically designed sleep recordings. When I was a kid, I loved having talk radio on in the background. Some people may even fall asleep to the noise of cars passing by their street. What about if they live in Manhattan? Honk, honk.

Cold Therapy

Many people claim to have changed their lives with cold therapy. This consists of getting into ice cold baths for a minute or two. Many say it calms the nervous system and I would say that is true. Will it reverse your sleeping issue alone? I doubt it. What it will do is help you through tough times as it helps with discipline.

Guided Recordings

Guided recordings could be great for you. Having a familiar voice to listen to over the course of ten to thirty minutes could knock you quick. That said, I have created a bunch of voice therapy albums for you. They're all available on spotify, apple music or youtube music.

Access yours: https://www.drkevinreese.com/voice

THE MEDICAL WAY

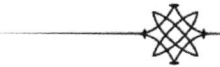

If you go to your primary care physician and tell them you're having trouble sleeping they are going to prescribe you some legal drugs.

The most common drug is Ambient (zolpidem). This drug is a sedative (hypnotic) that affects chemicals in the brain of people that may be unbalanced.

The side effects of Ambien may range from mild symptoms such as drowsiness to more severe symptoms like suicidal thoughts and significant next-day impairment.

Another bunch of legal drugs are benzodiazepines (benzos). These are depressant drugs which slow down the messages between the brain and the body. Benzos are typically used for anxiety cases but also can be prescribed for sleep deprivation. This includes Diazepam (Valium), Lorazepam (Ativan), Alprazolam (Xanax), Temazepam (Restoril), and Triazolam (Halcion).

Some side effects of benzos are short term memory loss, impaired thinking, irritability, slurred speech, headaches and more. If that's not bad enough, if you take benzos for a long period of time and then decide that you don't want them anymore, you will have to detox. It will not be fun or pretty and you could die.

If you continue to have sleep issues, the medical monopoly would love to refer you to a sleep clinic. Also known as polysomnograms, these clinics record your sleep patterns and activities. You'll wear sensors on your head, chest, legs, arms, and nose to measure your brain waves, eye movements, heart rate, breathing, and oxygen levels.

A technician will monitor you through the night from a nearby room, and you can talk to them if you need help. The study usually lasts 8–10 hours, and you can expect to receive your results within a few days. Sleep studies can help identify the cause of sleep problems and may lead to treatments like a CPAP machine or a mouth guard.

This is a great way for the Medical Monopoly to cash in some more.

SNORING & SLEEP APNEA

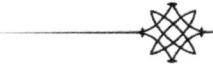

Snoring is a noisy, vibrating sound that occurs when air flows through the narrowed airway during sleep. It is caused by the relaxation of muscles in the throat and tongue, which allows the soft tissues to collapse and obstruct the airflow. Snoring can range from mild to loud and may be intermittent or continuous.

Snoring is basically harmless, but it is a symptom of a postural issue and or lymphatic stagnation in the head area. It can also be just the way you're laying. Certainly, PAT (postural alignment therapy) along with the proper nutrition can nip this in the bud.

Sleep apnea is a sleep disorder characterized by brief, repeated episodes of interrupted breathing during sleep. These interruptions, known as apneas, can last from a few seconds to several minutes and occur multiple times throughout the night. The Medical Monopoly claims that you can die from this condition and they prescribe a CPAP machine to wear for the rest of your life.

However, if you observe closely, you'll notice that babies and animals both technically have sleep apnea. Watch close. They hold their breath for long periods of time during sleep and sometimes make sudden movements.

You may also notice that you take shallow breaths during the day and then hold your breath unconsciously. Why? Because you tend to hold your breath when you overthink and or have high levels of concentration. The medical monopoly only tests you when you're sleeping, so how would they know about your breathing habits during the day?

While nutrition and mindfulness are involved in the condition they call Sleep Apnea, I feel it's mostly a postural issue. That means that your musculoskeletal system is out of alignment which is affecting your breathing. If you were to have a HEAD TO TOE ANALYSIS done, I think you would see how much your body is out of alignment and it would make sense to you.

Many of my students in my virtual learning membership stop using CPAP machines after a few months of PAT (postural alignment therapy). I'm happy to report that they're alive and well.

CANNABIS & CBD

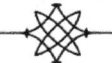

When marijuana (cannabis) became legalized everyone capitalized, including the sleep aid community. Many people use the marijana plant to sleep, some with success and some with no success.

The marijuana plant can be broken down into two categories of medicine. There is THC (tetrahydrocannabinol) and CBD (cannabidol).

THC supposedly increases slow-wave sleep, and increases total sleep time. Some people report feeling more focused and relaxed in the morning after using cannabis instead of sleep aids.

However, a 2022 study found that adults who used marijuana on 20 or more days in the past month were 64% more likely to sleep less than six hours a night. THC can also have side effects like anxiety and irritability.

Cannabidiol (CBD) may be a better sleep option than THC because it can reduce excessive daytime sleepiness. CBD may also help with PTSD, depression, c-monster, Parkinson's disease, multiple sclerosis (MS), and Alzheimer's dis-ease.

I feel like the marijuana plant has become like coffee because a million studies can say it's good and a million studies can say it's bad.

The overall common sense of the issue is that it's medicine. It's always been medicine, therefore, in my view, it's not something you want to take often. Same thing with all plant medicines, such as herbal formulas.

While cannabis is a better option than the medical monopoly's drugs, it's a moot point for my new health care system. If you're practicing HEAD TO TOE HEALING faithfully, then no medicine should be needed unless you have a birth defect, an infection or need a pain killer.

Again, HEAD TO TOE HEALING is made up of…

1-   Posture - The position of your musculoskeletal system.

2-   Nutrition - The raw materials that make up your body.

3-   Mindfulness - The management of stress and emotion.

PRIORITIZE YOUR SLEEP

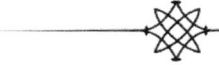

If you have friends and family, you're always going to receive peer pressure on your bedtime. Someone is always going to try and keep you up later. They will probably make a joke about it or call you "grandpa or grandma." It's ok. You do not need their approval. You are doing what is best for you. Your response should just be a joke sent back in their direction. You can say, "Hey, what can I say, it takes sleep to be this beautiful."

Perhaps no one gets hit with peer pressure more than the business owner. You see, regular people can't relate to a business owner. They view being a business owner as some privilege that has been bestowed upon them.

For example, if a business owner tries to leave the party early people say, "What? Why? You're the boss. You work for yourself. You can stay up." Meanwhile, when a regular person wants to leave the party all they need to say is, "Hey, I gotta go. I have to be at work at 6 AM" and everyone understands. Why? Because regular people can relate to getting up and "going to work." They don't take into consideration that the business owner's success may have been based on them getting up early!

Through the centuries, many great minds have gotten up early. Benjamin Franklin who is arguably the most productive and successful person of the modern era followed a strict schedule of going to bed at 10 PM and waking up at 5 AM. He used to say,

"Early to bed and early to rise, makes a man healthy, wealthy, and wise."

It's reported that Ludwig Van Beethoven slept from 10 PM to 6 AM, John Milton slept from 9 PM to 4 AM and Jeff Bezos says he sleeps from 9:30 PM to 5:30 AM. It's also been noted that many great minds may go to bed late but prioritize naps during the day. Albert Einstein slept for 10 hours per night and took naps. Some people need more sleep than others.

I tell my people all the time that health is your number one priority because without your health it's extremely difficult to be a productive member of society. Not to mention, it's harder to take care of your family and it's a challenge to enjoy life. Sleep is most certainly a major part of your health. This is how you recharge your batteries to take on another day.

It's difficult to be successful when you're walking around like a zombie. Lack of sleep also makes you vulnerable. While this vulnerability can open your heart, it tends to make you too emotional to handle life. This is evident with children. How many times have you seen a child crying and Mom says, "Awww someone needs a nap."

It's important to note that sleep is the time when your body heals. If you practice HEAD TO TOE HEALING, then all the work that you put in during the day will pay off while you're sleeping. Sleep is essentially the glue that holds together the three parts (postural alignment therapy, clinical nutrition and mindfulness training) of HEAD TO TOE HEALING. In other words, sleep is when you regenerate.

So what to do? You've already set your circadian rhythm to sleep from 10pm to 6am and your best friend wants to go out and stay up way past that time. Well, you have to decide if it's worth it. Yes, you're going to get made fun of, that's ok because you should not be worried about someone else's approval. Staying up until 2am when your body is used to going to sleep at 10am most certainly will have an impact on you the next day. So again, is it worth it?

The answer is relative. It depends on you. I personally feel that you should stick to your schedule but allow yourself grace to switch it up here and there. Perhaps it's new years eve or your wedding anniversary and you want to make your significant other happy. I say, as long as it's not all the time you're not making a huge concession.

Perhaps it can even be good mindfulness training to stay up late once per quarter. So the 4 times per year you stay up late, it's an opportunity to talk to your inner child (subconscious mind) and ease the worry. You can say...

"Baby, we are going to stay up late tonight because of the event we are going to. It's ok, don't be scared. I'm going to take care of everything and we are going to get great value out of this night. Tomorrow, we will take a little nap during the day and recharge ok? Then tomorrow night we will get back to our normal schedule. Everything will be ok. I love you."

BLUE BOOK BONUS

I created a series of voice therapy albums filled with meditations you can enjoy at your own convenience. There's one for sleep, one for easing anxiety, one for connecting with your future self, and more. I even recorded an entire album of bedtime stories, so you can go to sleep in peace.

Check it out: https://www.drkevinreese.com/voice

THE CHEAT CODE TO INNER PEACE

Many people don't sleep because they don't acknowledge that anything is wrong. Furthermore they don't accept the good, the bad and the ugliness of life. And lastly, they don't appreciate the ups and downs of their life's journey.

By living this way, you're creating resistance to life and resistance to life manifests into mental pain.

Some people don't even know that they are creating their own mental pain. They're just so frustrated, scared, guilty or full of grief that they go around in a vicious circle. Nothing can help them, including the legal drugs that the Medical Monopoly will put them on if they go see a white coat.

It's very hard to tell someone this.

It's like breaking bad news which can have some serious push back.

Truly I tell you, you don't have to suffer with mental pain. You can be mentally free.

What I am teaching you is a cheat code to inner peace. Think of it as a formula.

Acknowledgement + Acceptance + Appreciation = Inner Peace

Even if you don't have outer peace, you can most certainly have inner peace. So when you get triggered by something and you feel some mental pain, remember the cheat code.

When we are dealing with sleep troubles it's best to acknowledge you may have a problem. Then accept that you have this problem while using your discipline and courage to take action on fixing it. Then appreciate the lesson that is baked into the situation. You're being challenged.

REVERSE THE CAUSE

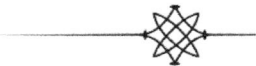

Here is a chapter from my book, REVERSE THE CAUSE that I wrote on Insomnia...

Insomnia is a common sleep disorder where you have trouble falling asleep, staying asleep, or getting good quality sleep. This happens even if you have the time and the right environment to sleep well.

Insomnia is arguably the worst condition there is. It turns you into a zombie. You walk around earth feeling like you're not human and your cognitive ability goes into the gutter. To make matters worse, you then become scared of not sleeping. During your day you'll say stuff to yourself like, "I hope I sleep tonight." This becomes almost like a PTSD.

If you go to the medical monopoly they will open up their treasure chest of legal drugs and give you a taste of hypnotic pharmaceuticals. These drugs may work for a few months, then your tolerance goes up. Then you're stuck.

Here are the root causes of insomnia from my head-to-toe healing perspective...

The first obvious root cause is nutrition. There's 90 essential nutrients that the body needs to import every day. That's 16 vitamins, 60 minerals, 12 aminos, and 2 EFAs. If you are deficient, your brain chemistry is thrown off. When it comes to sleeping, it's mostly deficiencies in the hard tissue category.

The second root cause is blood sugar imbalances which create inflammation. If you're not processing sugar properly, then the sugar is staying in your blood for too long of a time and it's creating inflammation. At the root this is nutritional deficiency because certain minerals are needed to process sugar. So if you're deficient and you keep eating and drinking sugar, you're in trouble.

Another root cause is going to be the mind-body syndrome (TMS). This is a lack of mindfulness where your negative thinking directly affects your body. Please understand that you have a computer in your skull. Your brain spits out data that operates in patterns or algorithms. If your computer is pumping out Michael Myers thoughts, then your frequency goes down and your body suffers. Keep in mind (no pun) that your brain is connected to your spine and your spine acts as a circuit breaker that sends electricity throughout the body.

When someone is caught in their head and worried about the future, they will have trouble sleeping. The biggest fear is death. Guess what sleeping is? It's a daily living death. You literally lose consciousness and pass out. Those that are scared to die subconsciously have trouble sleeping because of this fear.

Your environment certainly plays a factor with insomnia as well. The temperature and brightness of the room matter. Humans sleep better in a cold and dark room. Also, computer and phone screens can contribute. Too much screen time close to bed will throw you off.

Another reason for insomnia is when your routine is off. They call this the circadian rhythm. If you like to go to bed at 2am then your body will *want that. If you like to go to sleep at 9pm then your body will crave that. Going to bed at different times confuses your body.*

The most known root cause is going to be flat out pain. So many people come through my clinic who are miserable and it's just really hard to sleep. Back pain, knee pain, compressed nerves, lupus, diabetes, fibromyalgia, arthritis etc. Sometimes we have to get them feeling better before consistent sleep occurs.

I find that most people that have insomnia are just wound up too tight. They just care too much. It's a lack of acceptance of the good, bad and ugly parts of life.

FREE GOODWILL

It's been reported that people who help others with no expectation of anything in return experience higher levels of fulfillment. I'd like to create an opportunity to deliver this value to you during your reading or listening of this book. In order to do so, I have a simple question for you…

Would you help someone even if you never got credit for it?

If so, I have an "ask" to make.

There's someone out there in pain right now and they're confused and miserable. However, they don't know what to do about it and they don't know about my work.

The only way for me and my work to help people go from pain to peace is if this book has enough reach to get to their eyes and ears. People do actually judge a book by its cover but even more so, by their reviews!

So, if you've found this book valuable thus far, would you kindly take a moment right now to leave an honest review on Amazon and or Audible. It will cost you $0 and will take a minute.

Your honest review will help someone improve their life, which in turn, can help another person improve their life. We can create a ripple effect together. All you have to do is leave an honest review for any book of mine you read.

Thank you, I love you.

HEAD TO TOE HEALING

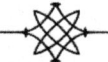

Fixing your sleeping issue is a big deal, but the practice of HEAD TO TOE HEALING is an even bigger deal. You see, sleep is just one part of health. There's so much more to it and if you don't get going on your journey, you could and will end up in a dark place.

The harsh reality is that the medical monopoly is not trained to heal you, they are trained to treat your symptoms, stabilize you and manage your pain with drugs, injections and surgeries.

In order to prove my new practice of HEAD TO TOE HEALING, I have captured the results on camera. People from all over the world on camera testifying to multiple symptoms disappearing.

This is confusing to many people because they have been brainwashed by the medical monopoly to need the help of specialists. You know, the spine specialist, the brain specialist, the GI specialist, the mental health specialist, the foot specialist and so on.

Well, my speciality is the whole body!

It's probably going to take another 100 years for people to truly understand HEAD TO TOE HEALING because people are so programmed to ask about their diabetes, or tinnitus, or bunions, or fibromyalgia, or migraines, or herniated disks etc that they lose sight of the truth.

The truth is…your body is a whole unit.

If there's something wrong with your feet, I want to see your ears. If there's something wrong with your ears, I want to see your feet. It's all connected.

HEAD TO TOE HEALING is the opposite of the medical monopoly specialist, it's about zooming out and viewing the body as a whole unit. Then we want to put it back into its natural alignment so that it heals. You see, the body is divinely designed to heal itself. God set it up this way!

To further understand how to perform HEAD TO TOE HEALING, I've broken the body down into 3 categories.

1. You have a vehicle (musculoskeletal system)

2. You need proper fuel for the vehicle (nutrition)

3. There's an onboard computer that runs the vehicle (the mind)

So if you have a pain in your left knee...

It could be coming from misalignments of your musculoskeletal system...

Or it could be coming from improper nutrition...

Or it could be coming from a lack of mindfulness...

It also could be coming from all three!

It doesn't matter because with the method of HEAD TO TOE HEALING, it's about getting after all three sections of the body, no matter what!

We approach type 2 diabetes the same way we approach a herniated disk, it's the same practice.

There's no over-diagnosis and there's no over-treatment with drugs, injections or surgeries.

You begin by ordering your HEAD TO TOE Analysis so that I can see the alignment of feet, knees, hips, shoulders, spine, neck and skull. Along with your nutritional profile and mental health status, you walk away with the root causes of your symptoms that a medical professional couldn't give you. This will give you the "ah-ha" moment that you needed to truly understand HEAD TO TOE HEALING. You also receive your "symptom score" which acts as a gauge to your health status.

Once you're evaluated and have a symptom score, you can enter my HEAD TO TOE HEALING Membership where you can come to our daily livestreams and start your 120 day program. This infamous program jumpstarts your HEAD TO TOE HEALING journey by getting after the whole body strategically.

So for example, if you scored a 30 on your analysis and your score at the end of 120 days is a 15, you're moving in the right direction. You're HEAD TO TOE HEALING.

Keep in mind, healing is a verb, it's a process, it's a moving thing which is why there can be no absolute "cure." Let the medical monopoly have the word "cure" we are HEAD TO TOE HEALING.

BLUE BOOK BONUS

I invite you to explore my YouTube channel, where I share longer videos—10 minutes or more—so I can explain things clearly and in depth. Be sure to subscribe, and leave a comment on one of the videos letting us know which book brought you there.

Check it out: https://www.youtube.com/@Dr.KevinReese

Q&A w/ Dr. Reese

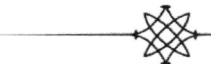

I'M ON STATIN DRUGS AND MY MUSCLES HURT. HOW DO I GET OFF THESE STUPID DRUGS!?

If I were you, I would simply just stop. Statins have no addictive quality to them and don't need a weaning process. If you'd like to play it safe, you can cut your dose in half for a few weeks and then stop. The reason you're having cramps is because the drugs have created a cholesterol deficiency in your body. Cholesterol is a very important nutrient that nourishes soft tissue. Muscle is soft tissue, organs are soft tissue, glands are soft tissue, eyes are soft tissue and most certainly, your brain is soft tissue. That's why most people that have been on statins for decades end up with dementia.

I HAVE TINNITUS? WHAT DO I DO? I'M GOING INSANE.

You do HEAD TO TOE HEALING. There's so many reasons why you could have this ringing in your ear that they call tinnitus. Is it the position of your neck? Is it a nutritional deficiency? Is it osteoporosis of the skull? Is it a blood sugar issue? The beautiful thing about HEAD TO TOE HEALING is it doesn't matter that much. You get after your whole body and let it do its work. Don't focus on the symptom, instead focus on your entire body. I suggest you order a HEAD TO TOE ANALYSIS and then get into the membership and you'll be on your way. If you view our testimonies, you'll see tinnitus disappear quite a few times.

IS THERE A CERTAIN WAY I SHOULD SLEEP SO I DON'T MESS UP MY POSTURE?

The answer is yes and no. Laying flat on your back is always the best way to rest. However, sleep is so important that you should sleep however you can. I would rather you get 8 hours in the fetal position than 3 hours on your back. So sleep however you can. This is why we do PAT (postural alignment therapy) in my membership. PAT is to your muscles what brushing and flossing is to your teeth. Your muscles need to be maintained daily. Also, as soon as you wake up, banging out some cats & dogs is ideal.

THEY TOOK MY GALLBLADDER! NOW WHAT?

Well, unfortunately, the medical monopoly doesn't tell you what to do. They just cut you and then sent you on your way right? So I'll tell you right now that you need to be on enzymes with ox bile for the rest of your life. You're now handicapped and need a crutch. I'll also tell you a harsh reality, you probably didn't need your gallbladder taken out. They are notorious for overdiagnosing. I have a course in my membership called Gallbladder Rescue that has helped many reverse their situation. Just know that the root causes that triggered your gallbladder are still there. It's like a shark circling the boat but you can't see the fin. You need HEAD TO TOE HEALING before more symptoms hit you.

I HEAR THAT ALL DISEASE COMES FROM THE GUT? IS IT TRUE?

No. This is a fun statement that health practitioners make because they are not HEAD TO TOE HEALERS yet. Certainly, the gut didn't cause your bunion or your herniated disk right? What they mean to say is that the gut is a root cause of most biochemical diseases. You see, muscle dysfunction is the root cause of most musculoskeletal misalignments (posture) which can also mess up the gut. Right in back of the gut is a spine and the position of that spine matters for gut health. Furthermore, the mind can give you gut symptoms. Understanding the body from HEAD TO TOE is a rare thing. Everything is connected.

HOW CAN I ORDER THE PROPER BLOOD LABS MYSELF WITHOUT MY PHYSICIAN? AND DOES INSURANCE COVER IT?

Inside my membership, we show you where to go, how to order and how to read the labs yourself. You can even order my recommended labs which cover most of your nutritional profile. Once you order, you can go to your local Quest or Labcorp to have the blood drawn and your results will be sent to your Quest or Labcorp phone app. It's not covered by insurance and that's a good thing. By paying out of pocket you are taking your control back and becoming independent. I'm teaching you how to save yourself and not be reliant on a corrupt system.

DR REESE, I'M SO DEPRESSED, I DON'T EVEN WANT TO GET UP IN THE MORNING. WHAT CAN I DO?

Make high pitched noises. Start there. This will elevate your frequency. Look at the word itself. It says that you're being pressed downward. So let's go upward! Furthermore, you need to make sure you don't have a nutritional deficiency. Missing one nutrient can cause up to 10 symptoms, so that's 900 total. Certainly, one of those symptoms could be depression. So getting on the right supplements is key. Of course, you have to get off the poor four foods (gluten, oils, friend and fake). You also could have a compressed nerve that alters your moods. However, the usual cause of depression is a lack of mindfulness. Many people get stuck in their heads and have a very negative voice talking in there. This creates disappointment and hopelessness. This is your inner child talking. In my membership, I teach my people how to work with the inner child to deprogram, reprogram and heal. The result will make you happy and appreciative.

WHAT TYPE OF WATER SHOULD I DRINK?

Well, not tap water. A RO (reverse osmosis) system is probably the most convenient way to filter water because once you install it you can drink it, cook with it, wash dishes with it and wash off food with it. Just make sure when you drink it, you re-mineralize. I also like the Berkey filtering system because it doubles as a mobile emergency unit. In other words, if your city's water becomes contaminated, you can find a local stream or pond and filter it through your Berkey unit. Hydrogen water is the new craze and it can help hydrate you perhaps better than any other water. As far as bottled water, it's best if you stay away from flimsy plastic because chemicals can leach into the water. Hard plastic is a better option and glass is the best option. Lastly, always stay away from carbonated and alkaline water, it decreases your stomach acid levels and will eventually cause acid reflux.

MY DENTIST SAYS I NEED A ROOT CANAL. SHOULD I GET IT DR. REESE?

If I were you, I wouldn't do it. There have been so many people who end up with health issues after this procedure. I have a course in my membership called Mouth Rescue. In there I will educate you on how to fix your mouth.

WHAT DO I DO ABOUT PARASITES?

Top off on stomach acid! Parasites only exist inside you if you don't have proper stomach acid (unless you're in a jungle). This is why so many vegans and plant based people have parasites. They detox out their worms and then show it off on social media which makes everyone paranoid that they have an infestation inside of them. The whole reason they had the worms in the first place is because they have low stomach acid and that acid is low because they've been obsessed with alkalizing. They're not HEAD TO

TOE HEALERS and don't understand the full scope of the body. You need a stomach acid level that is comparable to battery acid. Stomach acid deficiency is a root cause of a lot of symptoms, that's why we test it in our HEAD TO TOE Analysis.

WHERE ARE YOU LOCATED?

It doesn't matter. We are 100% virtual and help people from all over the world. We have people in my membership from the USA, UK, Australia, New Zealand, Portugal, South Africa and more. The only time to actually see me in person is at my annual seminar every spring. It's always held in my home state of Connecticut, USA. It's a great opportunity to not only meet me, but the rest of the membership. It's like a family reunion.

MY SISTER HAS AFIB AND IT'S DRIVING HER NUTS! WHAT CAN I DO TO HELP?

First off, you can't do anything except pass on information. She has to save herself. I would suggest MEDICAL MONOPOLY (red book) and HEAD-TO-TOE HEALING (green book). Give it to her and see if she wakes up. Please understand, AFib is typically a compressed nerve in the spine due to a musculoskeletal misalignment (posture). Then again, it could also be a nutritional deficiency. Does it matter? If your sister wakes up and does HEAD TO TO HEALING the chances of her AFib going away is very high.

SO YOU DON'T GO TO A DOCTOR?

I don't. I take care of myself through the practice of HEAD TO TOE HEALING. I pay out of pocket to run blood work once or twice per year just like I teach you in my membership. I do my PAT (postural alignment therapy), I take my supplements, I stay away from the poor four foods, I get 10,000 steps per day and I practice my mindfulness training. If something happens that requires medical attention, then I go to the nearest Urgent Care Center and pay a few hundred bucks. If something really serious happens, then I would use my health sharing program to pick up the tab for the ER. By not having a doctor I am claiming my freedom and adopting a HEAD TO TOE HEALING mindset. This is what I'm teaching you.

I HAVE FEET PAIN. WHAT SHOULD I DO?

Feet are at the mercy of your pelvis. When your pelvis is tilted, rotated or elevated it will affect the way you walk around earth (gait pattern). The more you walk a certain way the more your feet take a beating. Before you know it you may develop hammertoes, calluses or a bunion forming. We have a course in my membership called Foot Rescue that will move you in the right direction.

WHY DO YOU TALK SO SLOW AND WEIRD? IT'S CREEPY!

I'm working on different levels. One level I'm giving you health information so that you may heal yourself. On another level, I'm talking in a soft and calm way so that it may relax you from your busy life. On another level, I'm leaving space in between my words so that you can get to the spaciousness that's available to you. On another level, I'm putting out an energy that only those that are open can tap into. My style of communicating is not for everyone and that's good. If someone finds it creepy or weird, then I am not for them. They're not ready to be with me. Not everyone will understand what I have just said to you.

I AM ON 23 MEDICATIONS AND I FEEL TRAPPED!

You're in medical prison! This is the result of trusting in people that aren't trained to heal you. If you want to escape the prison, you have a long road ahead of you. If I were you, I would get off of any statin drugs or PPIs (proton pump inhibitors) because these are the two medications that are counteractive. In other words, you can't really perform HEAD TO TOE HEALING with them in your system. Next, get off the poor four foods (gluten, oils, fried and fake). Use my cookbook for recipes if you need to. Lastly, keep watching my videos. That's it. Start there because you're so programmed and traumatized right now that your inner child doesn't know who to trust! These three changes I just gave you will serve you well. Give it 60 days and I believe that you're going to feel major improvements. After you feel the changes and the faith has been established, come back and order an analysis. Then the next step is getting you into my membership and the journey of HEAD TO TOE HEALING will truly begin.

ARE YOU A KIND OF LIKE A CHIROPRACTOR?

No. Chiropractors are specialists in the alignment of the skeletal system. They snap, crackle and pop you with physical manipulation. In HEAD TO TOE HEALING we focus on the whole body (all 11 systems) and we don't have to lay a hand on you. That's how we have a virtual membership with people HEAD TO TOE HEALING from all over the world. People confuse me with a chiropractor because I'm talking about "alignment" all the time. The chiropractors kind of own that word just like the medical monopoly owns "diagnose," "treat" and "cure."

HOW DO I GET MY CHILDREN AWAY FROM THE HARMFUL JUNK FOODS?

Well, if they're under the age of 5 then I have a solution. I created a children's project based around a superhero named, SUNLIGHT SONNY. He flies all around the world helping kids stay away from the evil, Mr. Junkerson and his junk food. There's books, music and an animated TV show. However, if the kids are over 5, you have to just be repetitive and keep making them understand. A little trick you can pull if you're ok with a white lie, is telling your child that they're allergic to the poor 4 foods (gluten, oils, fried and fake). It works! I mean, most parents are already lying about Santa Clause anyway. You may be saving their future.

WHAT DO YOU THINK IS THE DISEASE THAT MOST AFFECTING SOCIETY?

Brain conditions, hands down. Everyone is scared of the C-Monster but it's dementia (Alzheimer's, FTD and Lewy body), parkinsons, ALS and MS that are making the biggest impact. How can we have a society when people's brains are compromised? A brain condition essentially takes you right out of the work force and puts you on the disability list. It's so preventable. It's a sad story.

WHAT DO YOU THINK OF THE CARNIVORE DIET?

I like the carnivore diet as a protocol. It's a great way to counteract conditions such as SIBO or Diabetes. However, I don't like the idea of being on this diet for longer than 90 days. Nutrition is based on ratios and all muscle meat is low in calcium and high in phosphorus which can trigger the body to steal calcium from the bones, teeth and nails. Therefore, someone that wanted to stay on Carnivore should be supplementing, as should everyone in the modern world. It's important to note that humans are meant to eat the whole animal, nose to tail, which would contain every nutrient needed. However, humans don't eat the whole animal anymore, they just like muscle meat.

I'VE SEEN YOUR ANALYSIS ON BRUCE LEE AND NOW I'M WORRIED THAT I ALSO MAY HAVE FORWARD HEAD. HOW CAN I FIND OUT?

First, thank you for paying attention to my videos. Second, in order to discover the position of your neck and head you would order a HEAD TO TOE Analysis. That way, I can evaluate your entire body, not just your head. Forward head, as you know now, is a problem in society. Once that neck starts falling out onto the chest, it's going to create "above the shoulder" symptoms. This could be ringing in the ears, dizziness, chronic headaches, eye issues, mouth issues and more. It could even contribute to dementia or parkinsons in the future. The reason why is because the lymphatic fluid in the head can't drain properly. Also, the blood and oxygen can't flow up to the brain, eyes, ears, nose and mouth as well.

SO YOU'RE SAYING I SHOULDN'T GET MY MAMMOGRAM?

If I were you, I would never have anything scanned unless I actually had symptoms (in this case a lump). Secondly, I would have it checked through Thermography. It's a very simple gray scan that can show lumps forming. It's important to note that if you do have a lump, you're still going to be faced with the medical monopolies only three solutions; drugs, injections or surgery. Perhaps I'm biased, but I feel that HEAD TO TOE HEALING is a better option due to the fact that the cause of the symptom(s) has to do with the whole body. The medical monopoly is just going to "zoom in" on the issue and throw the baby out with the bathwater.

HOW DO I BECOME AS CALM AS YOU DR. REESE?

It took me a very long time to evolve into the calm and peaceful man you see. Mindfulness training over and over and over again. It took a lot of failing. Luckily, I feel I have condensed the teachings and made it easier for you. You shouldn't have to go through as tough a time as I went through. In my membership, I'll teach you how to work with your inner child to move toward peace and healing. However, I do have a cheat code. It's the formula of acceptance + appreciation = inner peace. You see, most people have emotional imbalance because they don't accept life, therefore, they resist it in their head. They like the good of life but reject the bad and the ugly of life. Secondly, most people don't appreciate what they already have, including the hard times which are essentially lessons. For example, let's say you come out of the grocery store and your car window is smashed! What an inconvenience right? Well, accept it. Why wouldn't your window get smashed? It's a window! Also, appreciate that you even have a car to begin with. You know, some people take the bus. Also, appreciate the lesson that is being taught to you. Wait, what's the lesson? Find it, learn from it, smile, laugh and move on.

WAIT, YOU'RE NOT A MEDICAL DOCTOR?

That's correct. I'm a fake doctor. Dr. Reese is my stage name...kinda like Dr. Dre.

I HAVE HIGH CHOLESTEROL, WHAT SHOULD I DO TO CONTROL IT?

Nothing. In HEAD TO TOE HEALING, cholesterol is your friend and you don't want to try to control it. You need cholesterol to nourish your soft tissue. I would be more concerned with your Triglycerides and CRP levels as it pertains to cardiovascular health. You have been programmed to be scared of cholesterol, but it's not your enemy. You can read more about it in my book, REVERSE THE CAUSE and or there's a webinar I made for you on it on my website.

I HEAR ALOT ABOUT MOVING THE LYMPHATIC SYSTEM THESE DAYS. WHAT SAY YOU?

It's important. The lymphatic system is the sewage system of the body and it eliminates cellular waste from the body. Sometimes it can become clogged up from tight clothes, lack of exercise or from musculoskeletal misalignment. You want your lymph to be like a river and not like a pond. In my membership, we have three PAT (postural alignment therapy) classes per week. Not only will this get your musculoskeletal system back in alignment, but it will move your lymph. You see, the lymphatic system doesn't have a pump so it relies on your joints to act as a pumping system. You also need the "highways" to be open, so that's where something like tight clothes or muscle dysfunction slows things down. If the lymph slows down, many symptoms can occur, including tumors, nodules, cysts and polyps. In my membership, we also have a course called Lymph Rescue.

HOW CAN I MAKE AN APPOINTMENT WITH YOU DR. REESE?

I don't do personal appointments. Meeting with the "doctor" is an outdated strategy based on you feeling comfortable that an expert is there for you. I would rather you be uncomfortable and go on a journey to learn how to save yourself. If you're interested then go to www.DREKEVINREESE.com and poke around. When you're ready, make an appointment with my coaching team to see if HEAD TO TOE HEALING is the right fit for you. Remember, only you can save you.

WHY ARE OILS IN YOUR POOR FOUR FOODS? DO YOU JUST MEAN SEED OILS? THERE SEEMS TO BE SO MANY BENEFITS OF OLIVE OIL!

I teach my people to stop eating all oil, including olive oil. This is due to the fact that the oil has been pressed from the whole food. Now, this fat juice is vulnerable to oxidation from the air. Once that happens, the oil becomes rancid and free radicals are formed. Of course this creates free radical damage (oxidative stress) in the body which is a root cause for cardiovascular dis-ease and the C-Monster. If you go find a bottle of oil right now, you will notice space at the top of the bottle. In other words, the bottle isn't filled all the way up. What's in that space at the top? Right, it's oxygen. How long was the oil bathing in the oxygen? Hours? Days? Months? Now your salad is a weapon of mass destruction. Even worse, if you cook the oil, you've just made it even more destructive and you have set yourself up for a really ugly health event in the future. If you don't want to cook with water (that's how I cook) then use butter, ghee, lard or tallow like your ancestors did.

HAVING NO HEALTH INSURANCE SOUNDS SCARY, WHY ARE YOU RECOMMENDING THIS?

So that you can unplug from the medical monopoly and be independent. Of course it's a case by case thing. If you're stuck in MEDICAL PRISON then you have to have insurance. However, if you're a healthy person, why would you? Especially if you're practicing HEAD TO TOE HEALING. Consider this, a healthy person is going to pay more in premiums than if they got into an accident. Like I wrote in the book, they knock your cost way down if you tell them you do not have insurance. I personally like health sharing programs because they're somewhere in between. I pay $200 per month for my health sharing program. This covers me (they call it sharing) up to $1M in the event of an emergency. I have a course on all this in my virtual membership.

AFTER A SCAN ON MY SPINE, MY DOCTOR SAYS THAT I HAVE STENOSIS. CAN YOU TREAT THIS?

No. We do not treat anything. Treatment is a medical monopoly game. What we do is teach HEAD TO TOE HEALING so that you can get your body back into alignment so it can heal itself. Muscles move bones, therefore you don't have a spine issue, you have a muscle issue. Your muscles have bullied you and have pulled your spine in an odd direction that has created a narrowing which of course creates a slew of new symptoms. Furthermore, you have all sorts of nutritional deficiencies that are making the vertebrae and the cartilage weak. Now, based on my teachings, you have made a mistake. How? You went to the doctor and got tested. The more they test, the more they find. Now, it's stuck in your programming that you have a dis-ease called "stenosis" and that just sounds scary. What was the point? All they did was "zoom in" and look at a part of your spine instead of your muscles, feet, knees, hips, shoulders, neck, nutritional profile, stomach acid, mental health etc. Their solution is now going to be drugs, injections and surgeries, whereas in my membership, I'm teaching you HEAD TO TOE HEALING. It's your choice.

About The Author

Dr. Kevin Reese has helped thousands of people reclaim their health since 2010. He is the inventor of a new lifestyle practice called, HEAD TO TOE HEALING. This new approach to health has gathered the most healing results ever captured on video.

While he has a PhD in nutrition and a ton of certifications in other modalities, it's actually his self-study that made him different from everyone else. One day, Dr. Reese had an epiphany that the reason people aren't healing is that schools teach individual parts of the body. After this epiphany, he went on to study the brain, the spine, the pelvis, the gut, the blood, the lymph, the eyes, the feet, etc.

Learning how all parts connected with each other, he made the entire body his specialty and created HEAD TO TOE HEALING. He has authored 10 books on the topic including the best seller, MEDICAL MONOPOLY (the red book).

Through his videos, books and membership, Dr. Reese has attracted a passionate following of over a million social media followers along with fans that travel long distances to his speaking events to have their books signed.

Printed in Dunstable, United Kingdom